HAIR CARE BEGINS WITH YOU.

MONICA DE LA BASTIDE

ACKNOWLEDGEMENT

I acknowledge Anastasia De La Bastide for being an outstanding teacher and mentor. She made a significant impact on my life.

Anastasia was a true inspiration to me. She was always patient, kind, and willing to go above and beyond to help me learn and grow. Her dedication to her craft and passion for teaching was evident in every lesson she taught.

I will never forget the valuable lessons she imparted to me, memories we shared, and the impact she made on me. Anastasia's legacy as a great teacher and a wonderful mother will live forever in my heart and mind.

Thank you for everything.

CONTENT

INTRODUCTION

Hair care is an important aspect of our physical appearance and plays a significant role in our daily lives. Across cultures, hair is often considered a symbol of beauty and personality, and it can also be an indicator of overall health and well-being. Therefore, taking good care of our hair is essential for maintaining our health and vitality.

The importance of hair care goes beyond aesthetics, as proper hair care can minimize hair damage, loss, and other non-hereditary hair-related problems. A good hair care routine can improve the natural shine and strength of our hair, but it requires lots of attention, patience, and discipline. One's hair care routine or needs depend on their hair type and texture.

Basic hair care practices, such as washing and conditioning the hair, and regularly protecting it from unnecessary heat and environmental damage, apply to everyone. Additionally, maintaining a healthy diet can also promote healthier hair growth. It's important to note that the significance of hair care is not limited to women, as men should also care for their hair, especially if they are experiencing hair loss or balding issues.

In recent years, the hair care industry has grown exponentially, offering a wide range of products and treatments that are available to everyone. However, no single product or treatment is suitable for everyone, and it's crucial to understand the needs of your hair and choose products and treatments accordingly.

In summary, hair care is crucial for maintaining healthy and beautiful hair. By implementing a proper hair care routine, we can prevent hair damage, loss, and other hair-related problems, which can ultimately boost our self-esteem and well-being.

CHAPTER 1
UNDERSTANDING YOUR HAIR

THE STRUCTURE OF HAIR

Hair has a complex structure vital to our physical appearance and overall health. It consists of three parts, better known as layers, to each strand of hair: the cuticle, the cortex and the medulla.

The Cuticle:

The cuticle is the outermost layer of the hair made of overlapping cells, like shingles on a roof or the scales on a fish. The cuticle is the protector for the hair shaft. It also determines the shine and texture of the hair. Cuticles that lay smooth and flat give hair a shiny and healthy appearance. Damage cuticles cause the hair to appear frizzy and dull.

The Cortex:

The cortex is the middle layer of the hair. It gives the hair its strength, color and texture. The protein called keratin is found in the cortex and is responsible for the hair's structure and elasticity. The cortex also contains melanin, which gives the hair its natural color.

The Medulla:

The medulla is the innermost layer of the hair. It is a soft, spongy substance that runs down the center of the hair shaft. Not all hair has a medulla, and its function is still not fully understood.

THE GROWTH CYCLE OF HAIR

The hair growth cycle has three phases: the Anagen phase, the Catagen phase, and the Telogen phase.

The Anagen Phase:

The anagen phase is the active growth phase of the hair. During this phase, the hair follicle is actively producing hair. This phase can exist anywhere from two to six years.

The Catagen Phase:

The catagen phase is between the anagen phase and the telogen phase. During this phase, the hair follicle shrinks and detaches from the dermal papilla.

The Telogen Phase:

The telogen phase is the resting phase of the hair. In this phase, the hair follicle is inactive, and the hair is no longer growing. This phase lasts about three months before the hair falls out.

DIFFERENT HAIR TYPES AND THEIR CHARACTERISTICS

There are three main hair types: straight, wavy, and curly. Each hair type has its unique characteristics and requires different hair care techniques.

Straight Hair:

Straight hair is characterized by its smooth and sleek appearance. It is often thin and lacks volume. Straight hair appears shiny and healthy because of the natural oil flowing throughout the hair shaft. Therefore, it is necessary to cleanse the hair regularly.

Wavy Hair:

Wavy hair is loose curls and waves. It is thicker than straight hair and has more volume. Wavy hair tends to be dry and requires more moisture, use of moisturizing shampoo and conditioner.

Curly Hair:

Curly hair is characterized by its tight curls and spirals. It is often thicker than straight or wavy hair and has more volume. Curly hair tends to become dry and frizzy quickly, and it is better to use a moisturizing shampoo, conditioner and avoid heat-styling tools.

In conclusion, understanding the structure and growth cycle of hair is important. By knowing your hair's unique characteristics, you can choose the right hair care products and treatments to keep it healthy, shiny, and strong.

CHAPTER 2
HAIR CARE BASICS

Taking care of your hair is important. Hair requires the same essentials as a plant - nutrients, air, water, sunlight, love, and attention - to achieve a healthy, shiny, and strong head of hair.

Hair care tips that everyone could follow:

Cleanse:

Regularly shampooing your hair is essential for maintaining a healthy scalp and hair. It is safe to wash your hair 2-3 times a week, depending on the hair type.

Shampoo:

Choose a shampoo suitable for your hair type and scalp. Use a small amount of shampoo and massage it into your scalp and hair, focusing on the roots. Rinse thoroughly with lukewarm water.

Conditioning:

Conditioning helps restore moisture to the hair and prevents tangles and breakage. Always choose a conditioner suitable for your hair type and apply it to the mid-lengths and ends of your hair first. Leave it on for a few minutes before rinsing thoroughly.

Drying:

Towel-drying your hair can cause breakage and damage. Instead, use a microfiber towel or a t-shirt to squeeze out excess water. Avoid rubbing your hair with a towel. Allow your hair to air dry naturally or use a hair dryer to cool dry.

Brushing and combing:

Use a wide-tooth comb to detangle hair while wet. Avoid using a brush on hair that is porous, as it can cause breakage. Dry the hair completely before using styling tools.

Heat styling:

Excessive heat styling can cause damage to your hair. Heat styling tools should be used on hair after heat protectant spray or cream protect your hair from damage. Avoid high heat settings and limit heat styling to once or twice weekly.

Protecting your hair:

Protect your hair from environmental damage by wearing a hat or a scarf when you are in the sun. Hot tools on wet hair can cause damage. As a precautionary measure, avoid pulling your hair too tightly when styling it, as it can cause breakage and damage.

Nutrition:

A healthy diet is essential for maintaining healthy hair. Prepare foods rich in vitamins and minerals, such as fruits, vegetables, whole grains and lean proteins. Drink plenty of water to keep your hair hydrated.

In conclusion, following these hair care tips can help you maintain healthy hair. By understanding your hair type and its unique characteristics, you could choose the right hair care products and treatments to keep your hair looking and feeling its best. Always be gentle with your hair and avoid excessive heat styling and harsh chemicals.

CHAPTER 3
HAIR STYLING

DO'S AND DON'TS OF HAIR STYLING

When it comes to hair styling, there are certain dos and don'ts that you should keep in mind to keep your hair healthy and looking its best.

DO'S:

- Use heat styling tools in low to medium heat settings to avoid irreversible damage to your hair.

- Use a heat protectant spray or cream before using hot-styling tools.

- Use a wide-tooth comb to comb through wet hair to prevent breakage.

- Experiment with different hairstyles and hair accessories to find what works best for you and your hair type.

- Use hair products, such as hairspray or hair gel, sparingly to avoid buildup and potential damage.

- Use natural hair oils such as coconut or argan oil to nourish and hydrate your hair and scalp.
- Protect your hair from environmental damage by wearing a hat or scarf.
- Get regular trims to prevent split ends and promote healthy hair growth.

DON'TS:

- Don't use heat styling tools on wet hair.
- Don't use harsh chemicals such as bleach or ammonia on your hair.
- Don't pull your hair too tightly when styling.
- Don't brush your hair when wet.
- Don't use hair elastics with metal clasps, as they can snag and break your hair.
- Don't use an abnormal amount of product, as this may create buildup.
- Don't use hot tools on the same section of hair for too long, as this can cause damage and breakage.

In conclusion, protect your hair from damage and keep it looking healthy and beautiful. Remember to be gentle with your hair and avoid excessive heat styling, harsh chemicals, and tight hairstyles.

Implementing this will promote healthy hair growth and maintain a luscious head of hair.

CHAPTER 4
THE DIFFERENT TREATMENTS AND THEIR BENEFITS

There are many different hair treatments available that offer a range of benefits for your hair.

Here are some of the most popular types of hair treatments, along with their benefits:

Deep Conditioning:

Deep conditioning treatments penetrate the hair shaft and provide moisture and nourishment to dry or damaged hair. They can help restore elasticity, reduce breakage, and improve the health and appearance of your hair.

Protein Treatments:

Protein treatments help strengthen, and repair hair damaged by chemical or heat styling. They contain protein-rich ingredients that help to rebuild the hair's structure and improve its strength and resilience.

Keratin Treatments:

Keratin strengthens the hair while adding shine and reducing frizz. Keratin creates a protective layer around each strand.

Scalp Treatments:

Scalp treatments address scalp issues: dryness, dandruff, or irritation. They can help to soothe and hydrate the scalp, promote healthy hair growth, and improve the overall health of your hair.

Hair Masks:

Hair masks are similar to deep conditioning treatments but thicker and more concentrated. They are designed to provide intense hydration and nourishment to the hair and can help repair hair and reduce frizz.

Each type of hair treatment offers unique benefits, and choosing the best treatment depends on your hair type and specific concerns. Regular use of hair treatments can help improve the health and appearance of hair and can be a part of a comprehensive hair care routine.

WHY USING HOT OIL TREATMENT?

Hot oil treatments can be beneficial for dry or damaged hair. If the hair feels brittle, weak, or lacking moisture, a hot oil treatment can help to restore shine and softness. The heat from the oil also helps to open up the hair cuticle, allowing the oil to penetrate more deeply and provide maximum benefits.

There are several ways to do a hot oil treatment at home. One method is to warm up your preferred oil in a bowl of hot water, then apply the oil to your hair and scalp by following the direction for that product. You can then wrap your hair in a warm towel, Saran wrap, or shower cap and leave the oil on for 30 minutes or as directed. Another method is to apply the oil to the hair and scalp, then use a hair dryer to heat the oil for a few minutes or a heating cap.

Hot oil treatments can be done once a week or as needed, depending on the hair's condition. Extremely dry or damaged hair may require hot oil treatment more frequently to help restore moisture and strength. Hot oil treatments can be a great addition to the hair care routine.

DIY HAIR MASK

Here is an example of a DIY hair mask that you can make at home using natural ingredients:

Avocado oil and honey hair mask:

Ingredients:

- 8Tablespoons Avocado oil
- 2Tablespoons honey

Instructions:

- Heat the avocado oil on the stove until it is melted and warm.

- Add the honey to the oil and stir until the two ingredients are well combined.

- Apply the mixture to damp hair, starting at the roots and working down the hair shaft to the ends.

- Use your fingers to massage the mask onto your scalp and hair, covering the entire head of your hair.

- Cover your hair with a shower cap, Saran wrap, or warm towel for at least 30 minutes.

- Rinse the mask out of your hair with warm water, followed by mild shampoo and conditioner as usual.

This hair mask adds moisture and shines to dry or damaged hair. Coconut oil is rich in fatty acids that help to nourish and hydrate the hair. Coconut oil is known for its help in the fight against fungus. Honey is a natural humectant that helps to lock in moisture. Customize this mask by adding ingredients, such as avocado or aloe vera, to suit your hair's specific needs.

CHAPTER 5

HAIR CARE FOR SPECIFIC HAIR TYPES

air comes in various types, and each type has its unique characteristics and challenges. Understanding your hair type and how to care for it can make a significant difference in achieving healthy, strong, and beautiful hair.

HAIR TYPES AND TIPS

Straight Hair:

Straight hair tends to be oilier and can become weighed down.

Tips

A mild shampoo and conditioner will avoid stripping the hair of natural oils. Avoid heavy styling products hair may appear greasy and flat. For added volume, use a dry shampoo or texturizing spray. Consider the backcombing method that creates the appearance of a fuller head of hair.

Wavy Hair:

Wavy hair can be prone to frizz and tangles. Therefore, a moisturizing shampoo and conditioner will keep your hair hydrated and detangle-free.

Tips

Try using a leave-in conditioner or styling cream to help define your waves and keep them looking smooth.

Curly Hair:

Curly hair tends to be drier and more prone to damage than other hair types.

Tips

Use a sulfate-free shampoo and conditioner to avoid drying out your hair further. Apply a leave-in conditioner or styling cream to help define your curls and prevent frizz. The best way to enhance your curls is to blow dry your hair using a diffuser.

Tightly Curl Hair:

Tightly curled hair is known for its elasticity and naturally dry appearance, leaving it prone to breakage.

Tips

Use a moisturizing shampoo and conditioner to help keep your hair hydrated. Apply a leave-in conditioner to help seal in moisture and prevent breakage. Avoid using heating tools.

Fine Hair:

Fine hair can be prone to limpness and flatness.

Tips

Use shampoo and conditioner that increases volume by adding body and fullness to your hair. Add a mousse or volumizing spray to add more volume to your hair.

In conclusion, avoid heavy styling products, as they can weigh your hair down and make it appear flat. Do not be afraid to experiment with different products and styles to find what works best for you.

CHAPTER 6

HAIR PROBLEMS AND SOLUTIONS

Hair problems can range from hair loss to dryness, but with the right hair care regimen and treatments, these issues can be resolved.

Common Hair Problems and Their Solution

1. **Dryness and brittle hair:**

Dry hair is due to a lack of moisture in the hair caused by poor dietary practice, over-washing, using harsh shampoos, using heat styling tools frequently, or excessive exposure to the elements such as sun and wind.

SOLUTION

- Use a moisturizing shampoo and conditioner.
- Deep treatment once a week could help add moisture to your hair.
- Use less heat styling tools and protect your hair from the sun and wind.

2. Split Ends:

Split ends occur when the ends of the hair split apart. The hair is like a flower, and it is in its blooming phase. Although heat-styling tools, exposure to the sun and wind, and using harsh hair products cause damage. This natural occurrence takes place during the spring season more than any other.

SOLUTION

- The only solution to split ends is to trim them off.
- Trimming off split ends: one to three inches of hair should be removed.
- Regular haircuts can help prevent split ends from occurring.

3. Dandruff:

Dandruff is dead skin cells on the scalp, dry scalp, oily-overactive sebaceous glands, and hair products are the leading contributor.

SOLUTION

To eliminate dandruff, use a medicated shampoo specifically for fighting dandruff. A dermatologist narrows the choice of dandruff shampoo to one that will provide the best results in a shorter time frame. Massage the shampoo into your scalp and leave it on as described or directed by a dermatologist.

4. Hair Loss:

Hair loss causes may vary, including genetics, hormonal changes, stress, the tension on the follicle, and illness.

SOLUTION

- A healthy diet and lifestyle are the first step when dealing with hair loss.
- Use hair products for sensitive skin and avoid tight hairstyles that may put tension on hair follicles.
- Consider using a hair growth treatment recommended by your dermatologist to help promote hair growth.

5. Oily Hair:

Oily hair is a result of an overly active sebaceous gland, genetics, hormonal changes, or using heavy hair products.

SOLUTION

To combat greasy hair, shampoo with a product specifically designed for oily hair. Reduce shampoos to slow down excess oil production. One of the benefits of dry shampoo is; absorbing excess oil

In conclusion, common hair problems and their solutions can help keep your hair healthy and beautiful. If you are experiencing persistent hair problems, consult a dermatologist or hair care professional for personalized advice.

CHAPTER 7

HAIR CARE FOR MEN

Taking care of your hair is important, and men can benefit from a hair care system designed specifically for their unique hair and scalp needs.

A Hair Care System for Men

Shampoo:

Selecting a shampoo that addresses your haircare needs, such as dandruff, oily scalp, or thinning hair, apply shampoo to the scalp and massage it gently into your scalp with your fingertips for a few minutes before rinsing it out. Follow directions for best results.

Conditioner:

Conditioners nourish and moisturize your hair, making it soft and more manageable conditioners should provide the benefit required to accomplish the desired result.

Styling products:

Pick styling products designed for men's hair gels, pomades, waxes, or sprays, and use them sparingly to avoid weighing down the hair.

Regular haircuts:

Regular haircuts are essential for a men's hair care system on average every 2-4 weeks or as often as necessary to maintain your desired style.

Scalp care:

Massage the scalp daily to increase blood flow to hair follicles.

TIPS ON MALE BALDING OR THINNING HAIR

Hair loss is difficult for men, experiencing significant hair loss or thinning hair may require medical attention to determine the root cause of your hair loss and suggest appropriate treatment options.

TIPS

- **Consider medication:** Several medications help to slow or even reverse hair loss in some men. A physician can prescribe medications that promote hair growth and prevent further hair loss.

- **Be gentle with your hair:** Avoid rough handling of your hair, including excessive brushing, combing, or styling, wash your hair, and avoid using hot water or harsh shampoos that may create further damage to hair and scalp.

- **Use hair products with care:** choose hair products that are gentle and avoid harsh chemicals that can further damage your hair and avoid products that coat the hair.

- **Consider a new hairstyle**: A new haircut or hairstyle can help conceal thinning hair and the bald area. Style should complement your hair type and facial structure.

- **Practice good scalp care:** Keep your scalp healthy by washing it regularly and using a scalp scrub or serum to promote circulation while delivering nutrients to the hair follicle scalp massaging brush can stimulate hair growth and improve blood flow to your scalp.
- **Embrace baldness:** If your hair loss is significant, you may want to consider embracing baldness men that shave their heads or opt for a buzz cut find it liberating and empowering.

CONCLUSION
RECAP OF TOPICS COVERED

- Hair types: Understanding your hair type is essential for developing a hair care routine that works best for you.

- Type of hair includes straight, curly, wavy, and tightly curled. Each hair type may require different care.

- Shampooing and conditioning: Regular shampooing and conditioning of hair leave the scalp free from buildup work with a product brand appropriate for your hair type.

- Styling: use simple styling techniques and avoid heat-styling tools as much as possible to prevent damage.

- Diet and lifestyle: A healthy diet and lifestyle play a significant part in the health of your hair.

- Hair loss: Hair loss is a common issue affecting many people, and treatments are available, based on the cause of the hair loss, to help promote hair growth and prevent further loss.

FINAL TIPS FOR HEALTHY HAIR CARE

- Avoid using hot water when washing your hair.
- Use a wide-toothed comb to detangle your hair.
- Avoid using harsh chemicals on your hair.
- Avoid tying your hair tightly.
- Protect your hair from the sun and other environmental factors.
- Get regular haircuts to maintain healthy hair.
- Use hair masks and other treatments to nourish and protect your hair.
- Hair average growth is half an inch per month.

FINAL RECAP ON HOW TO TAKE CARE OF YOUR HAIR:

- Keep your hair clean:
- Cleanse your hair regularly with a mild shampoo to remove dirt and excess oil.
- Rinse with lukewarm water.
- Hot water will strip your hair of its natural oils.
- Condition your hair: After shampooing, use a conditioner to keep your hair moisturized and soft. Apply it to the ends of your hair and work your way up to the roots.
- The use of hair oil: Apply hair oil to the scalp to nourish and strengthen your hair.
- Massaging your scalp after applying oil can also improve blood circulation and promote hair growth.
- Limit dry heat styling: Heat styling tools like flat irons and curling irons can damage your hair.
- Always apply heat protectant before using hot tools.
- Protect your hair from the sun: Exposure to the sun can damage hair and cause it to

become dry and brittle, use a leave-in conditioner with SPF protection.

- Tight hairstyles: Tight hairstyles like braids, buns, and ponytails can pull on your hair and cause breakage and weak hair follicles.
- Wear loose styles whenever possible.
- Trim your hair regularly: Regular trims can help prevent split ends and stimulate the flow of natural hair oil through the hair shaft.
- Eat a healthy diet: A diet rich in vitamins and minerals can help keep your hair healthy, such as eggs, nuts, beans, and green leafy vegetables.

By following these tips, you can keep your hair healthy. Everyone's hair is unique, so experiment with different products and techniques to find what suits your hair type and what works best for you.

Copyright © 2023/ MONICA DE LA BASTIDE.

ABOUT THE AUTHOR

Monica De La Bastide is known for her creative abilities as a Cosmetologist and her caring nature which helped her to stand out during those years as a hairstylist and business owner. Hair health is her passion.

She started her journey in the beauty industry due to her curiosity. That interest in the transformation of one's appearance became more interesting as the years rolled by.

She got her first taste of Entrepreneurship at the age of seven and she never looked back. Being a proud mother to three beautiful children and the firstborn child for parents she is embarking on something greater, generational expansion, to be recognized as a successful Inventor.

LET'S STAY IN TOUCH!

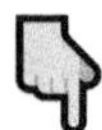

Visit my website @
https://haircarebeginswithyou.com/

You can as well subscribe to my newsletter @
https://haircarebeginswithyou.com/newsletters/

or send a direct mail to me @
info@haircarebeginswithyou@gmail.com

I can't wait to hear from you!

www.ingramcontent.com/pod-product-compliance
Lightning Source LLC
Chambersburg PA
CBHW050752250726

48662CB00005B/2182